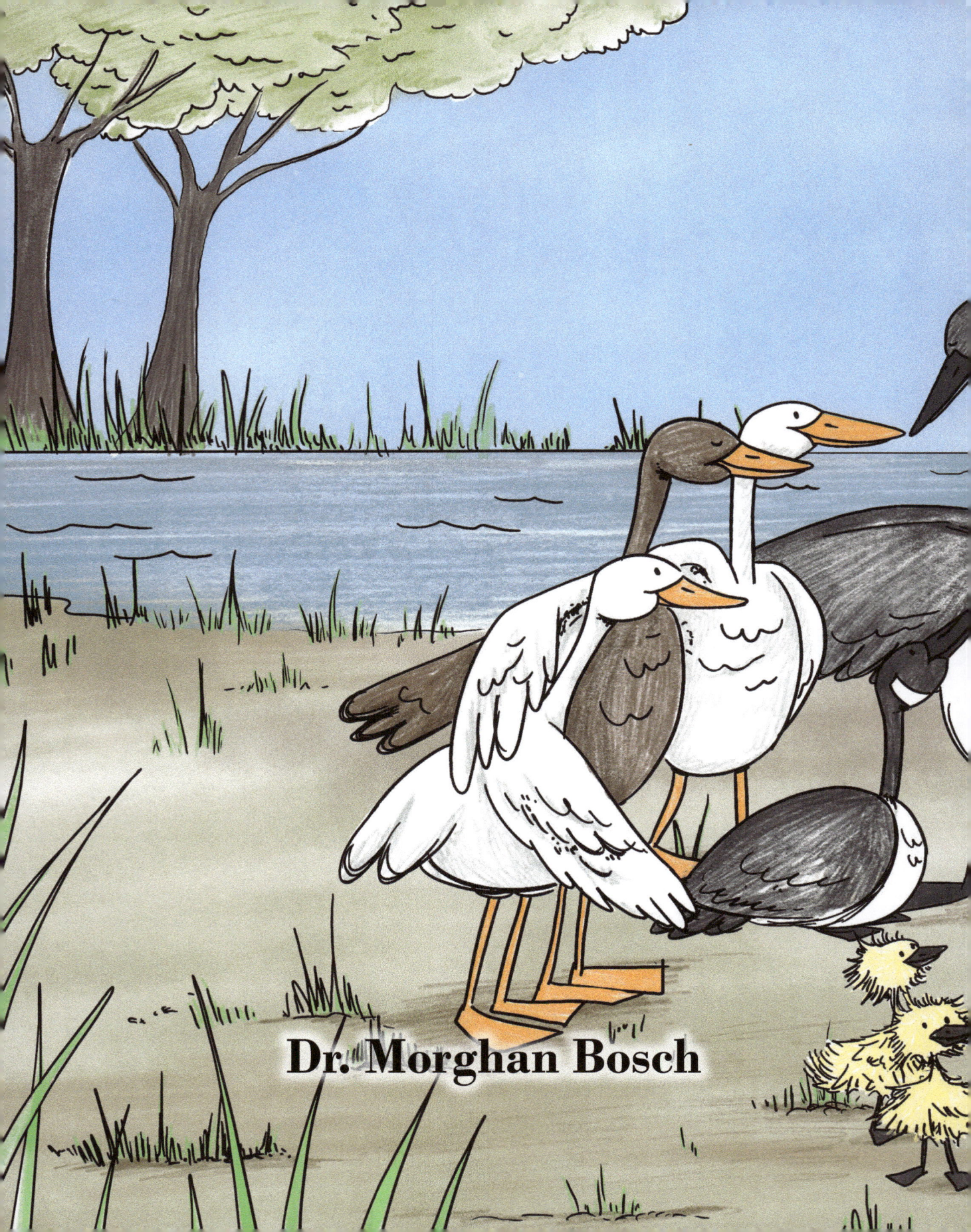

Dr. Morghan Bosch

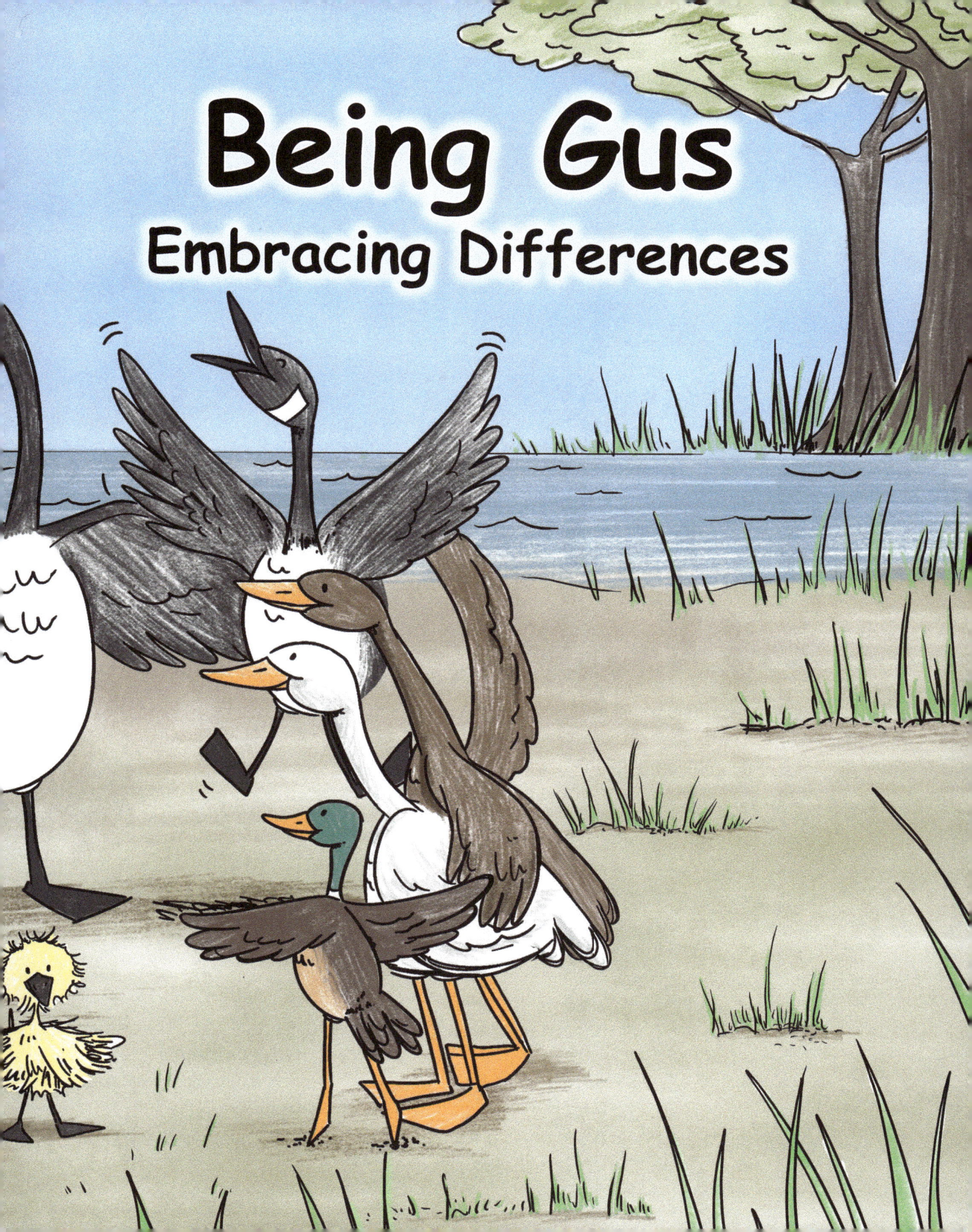

Being Gus
Embracing Differences

ISBN 978-1-63885-852-2 (Paperback)
ISBN 978-1-63885-853-9 (Digital)

Covenant Books
11661 Hwy 707
Murrells Inlet, SC 29576
www.covenantbooks.com

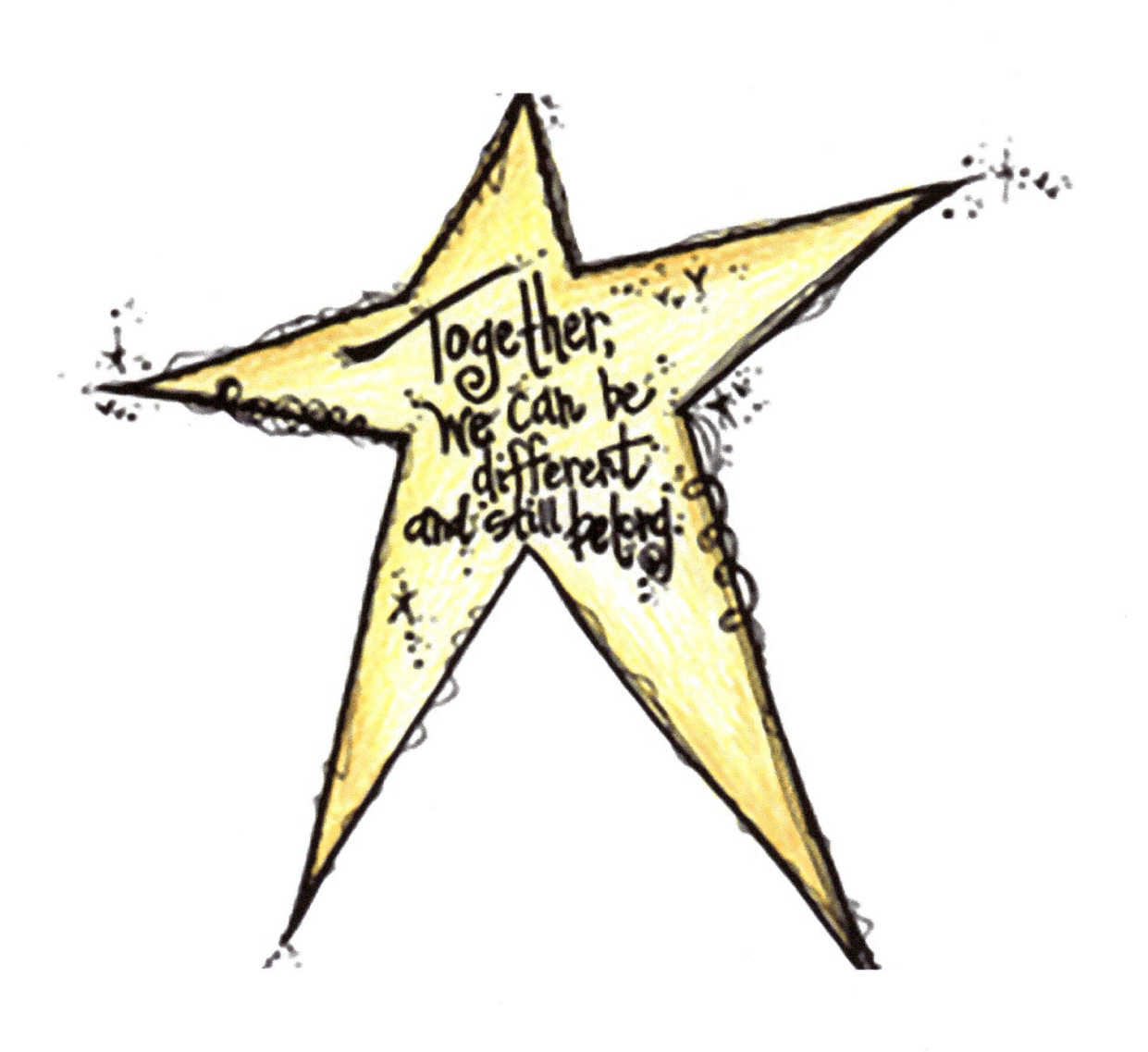

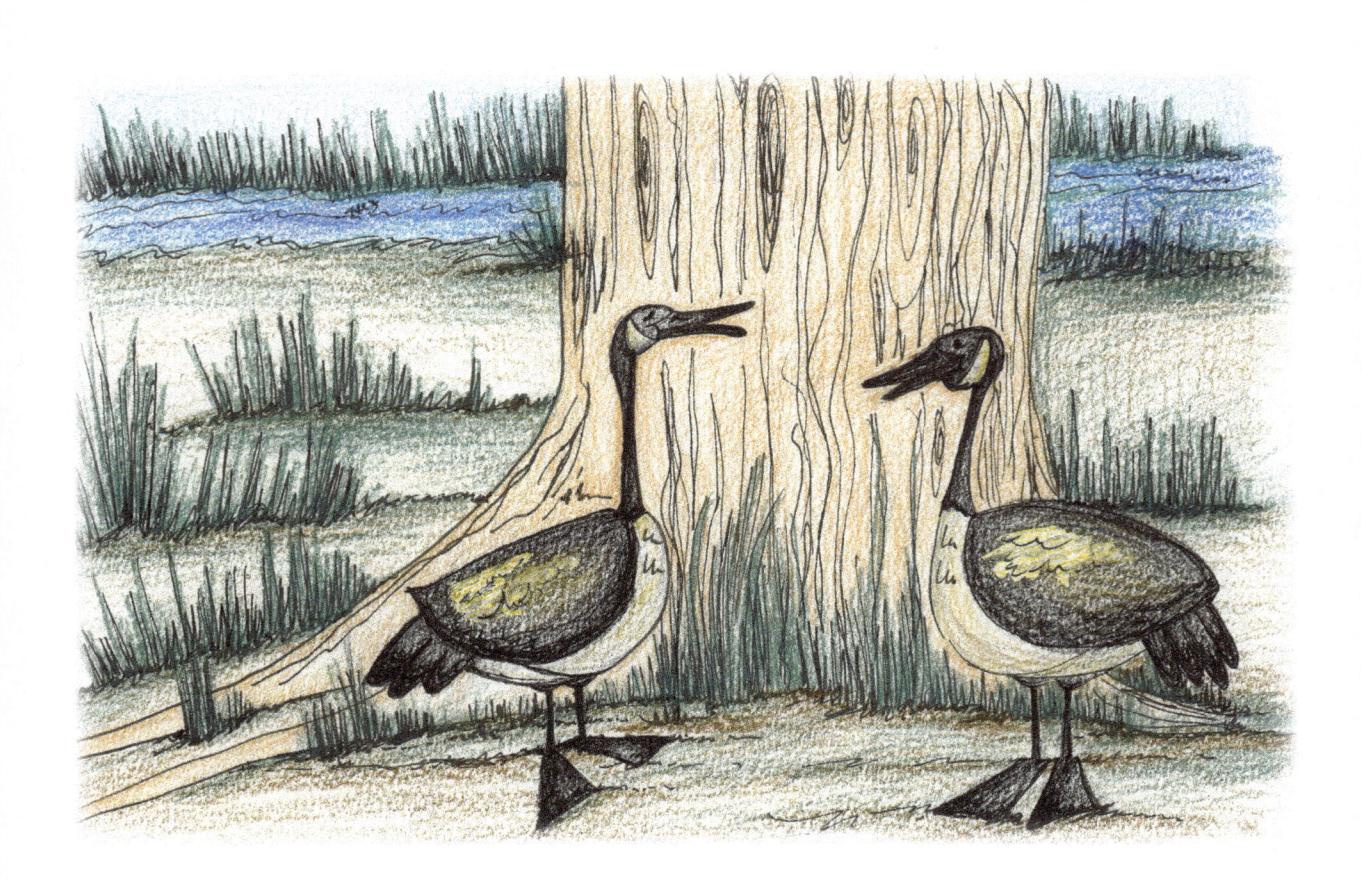

Prologue

This is the second book, *Being Gus: Embracing Differences*, in the series *Embracing Differences*. The first book was *Being Charley: Embracing Differences*. Charley was unlike his siblings; he had autism. Each book in the series will be about Charley's siblings. You have met Gus in the first book, and now you will get to know him even better.

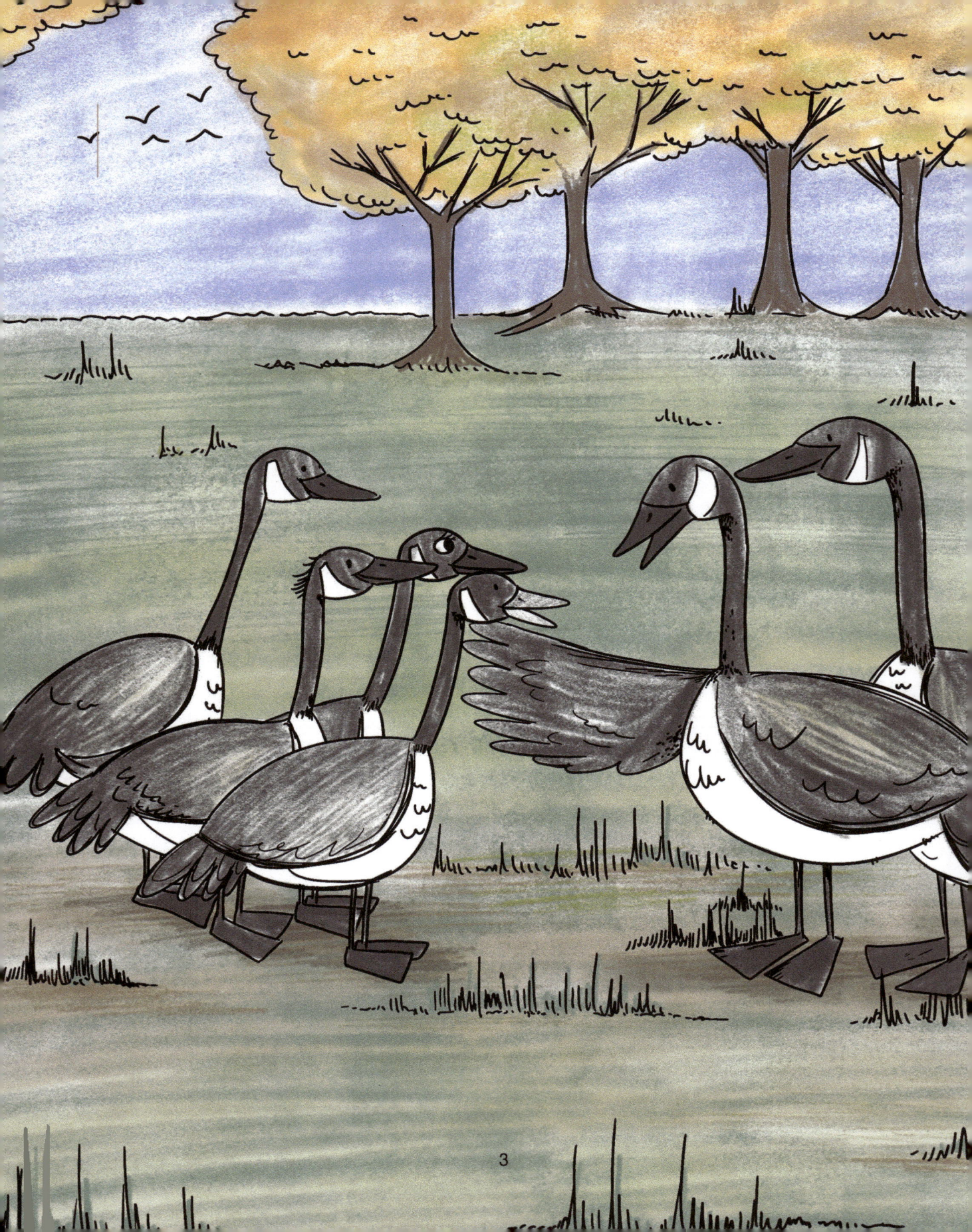

There was a chill in the air. Across the sky, the *V* formations of Canada geese were seen. They were traveling south to their wintering grounds.

Canada geese learn the migration routes from their parents and follow the same routes year after year. They even stop at the same rest areas.

As evening approached, Mama Goose gathered the family flock together. She announced, "In the morning we will begin the flight to our wintering grounds." The siblings Gus, Josie, Gertie, and Sammy were so excited because that meant they would visit Charley.

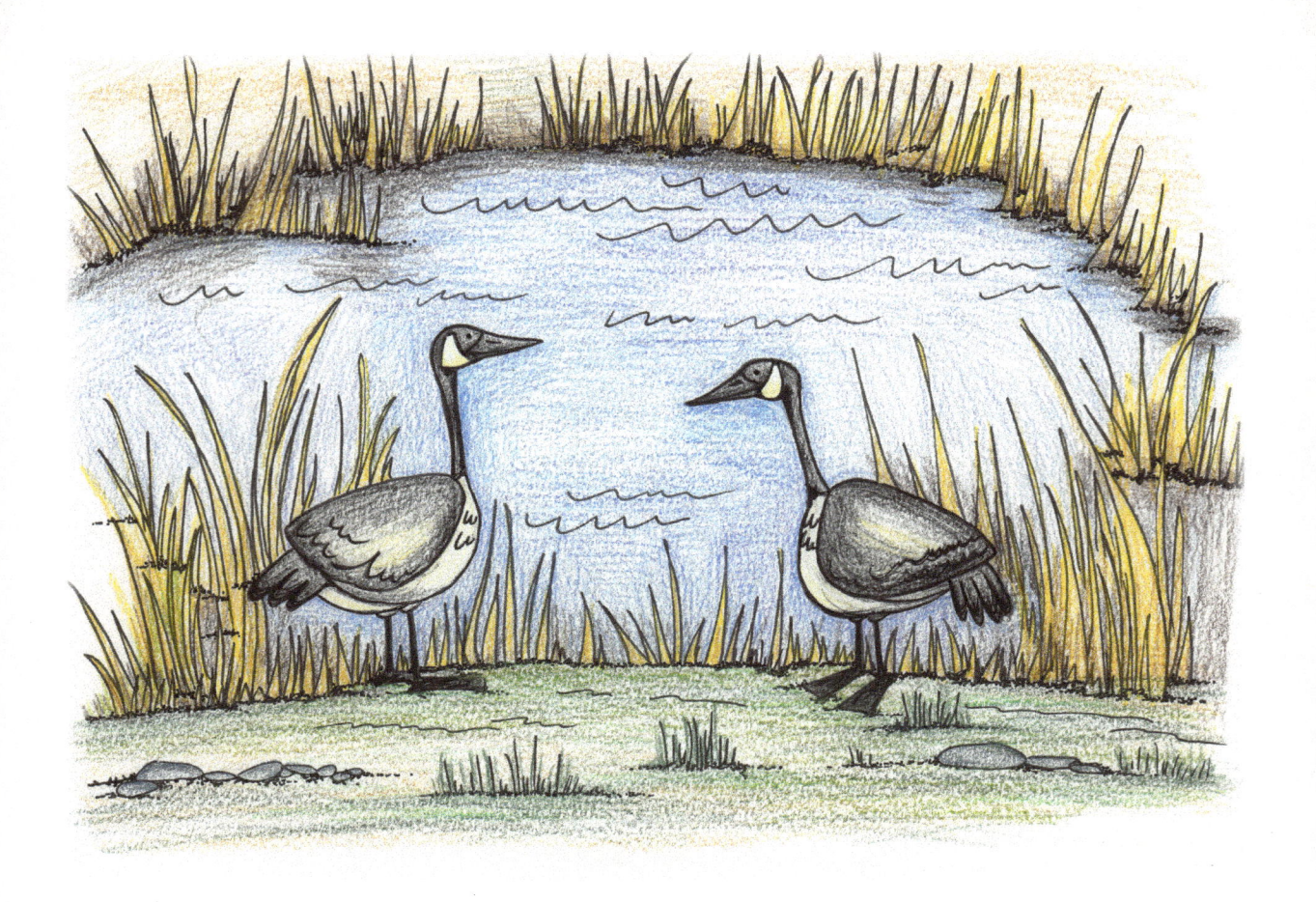

Mama Goose knew Gus worried about Charley. Gus was a caregiver and Charley's big brother, and she had asked Gus many times to watch over Charley. Gus looked at Mama Goose and said, "I miss caring for Charley. I enjoyed taking Charley to his quiet place. I listened to Charley's thoughts and fears. Many times, when Charley could not sleep, we would talk well into the night." Gus had a secret he was not telling anyone. He was planning to not only visit Charley but to stay with him at his place.

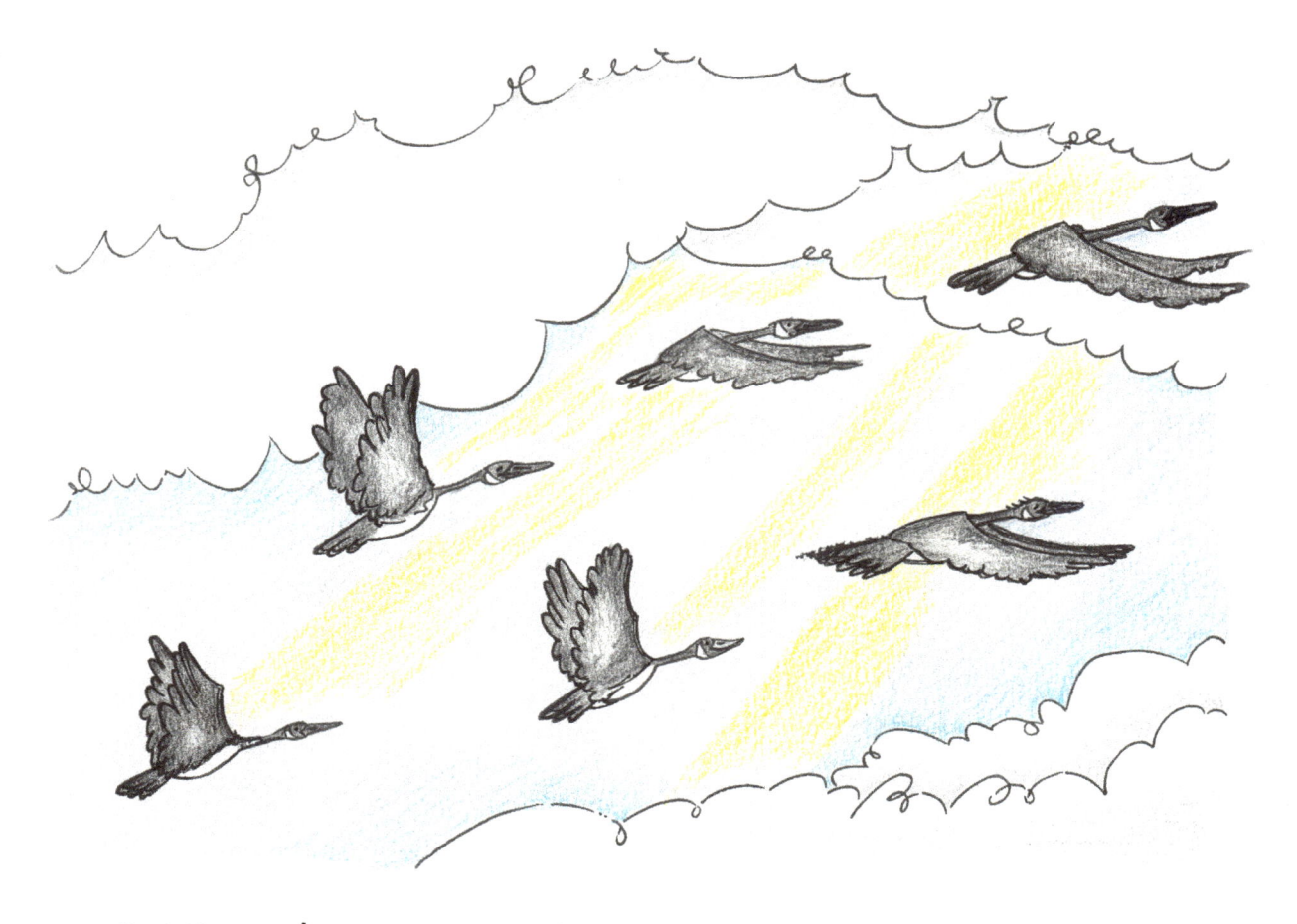

Getting a late start in the morning because the weather was very windy, the family flock took flight. Father Goose started as the leader with the rest of the family following in the V formation.

The geese take turns being the leader. When one tires, another goose takes its place as the leader of the V formation.

They flew a few days and soon reached Charley's place. The family flock circled overhead and landed close to Charley and his friends. Mama Goose and Father Goose and the siblings honked loudly and surrounded Charley and his friends. They were so loud Charley had to cover his ears. Gus sensed Charley's discomfort and quickly quieted everyone's honking.

With nightfall, Charley took the family flock and his friends to a special area by the pond. He wanted to tell them more about the night sky. He explained that the Big Dipper looked like a pot with a handle and had seven bright stars. Charley asked, "Did you know the Big Dipper changes its location from season to season?" He continued by explaining that the location of the Big Dipper was low in the sky in the fall and winter and high overhead in the spring and summer. The shape of the Big Dipper changes from upright to sideways to upside down with each season.

Charley said, "Because it is fall, look for the Big Dipper low in the sky, and it is shaped like a pot with a handle ready for the stove."

Josie suddenly exclaimed, "I see it! I see the Big Dipper with seven stars!"

Gus glanced over to Charley and secretly gave him a wings-up.

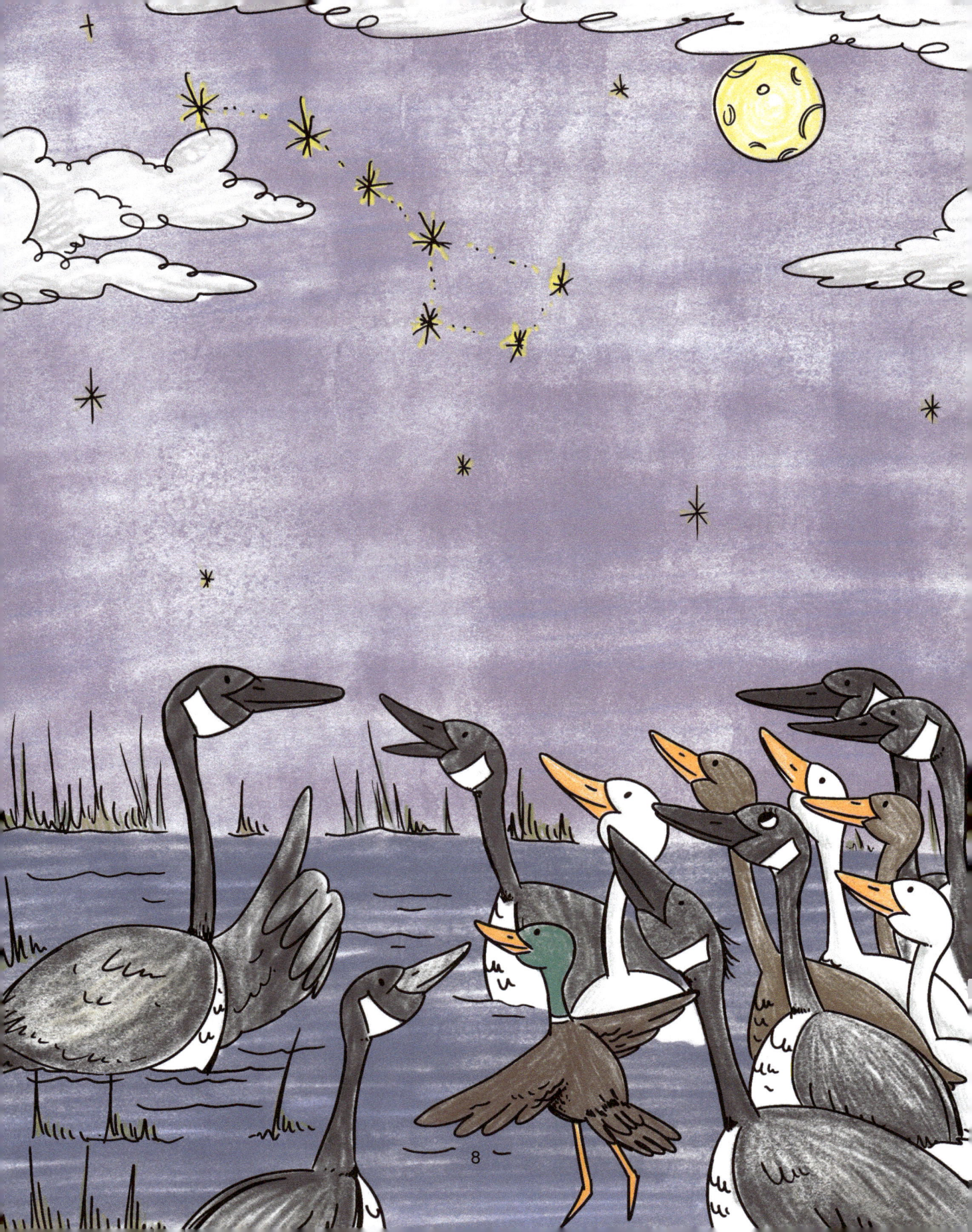

8

The family flock stayed at Charley's place for a couple of days visiting. One evening, Mama Goose gathered the family flock together to remind them they were leaving the next day. Mama Goose and Father Goose asked Charley if he wanted to join the family flock. Charley looked at Mama Goose and Father Goose and then at Gus and said, "I love you all and miss you, but this is my home." Gus, nervously, knew the time had come to tell everyone his secret.

Gus honked loudly to get everyone's attention. They all turned around and looked at him and wondered what was going on. He sputtered and finally said, "I am not flying to the wintering grounds with the family. I am staying here with Charley. I am his big brother, and I want to be with him."

The family flock stared at Gus with shock. Gus knew Mama Goose would miss him. Father Goose, beaming with pride, walked over to Gus and shook wings with him and wished him well. Everyone gave Gus a family hug. Gertie reminded her siblings, "Now we will see both Charley and Gus each time we migrate."

Charley was surprised. He could not believe what he heard. No one knew that Charley wished on a star every night that Gus would join him. He missed his big brother so much. His wish had been granted. Gus and Charley would be together from now on.

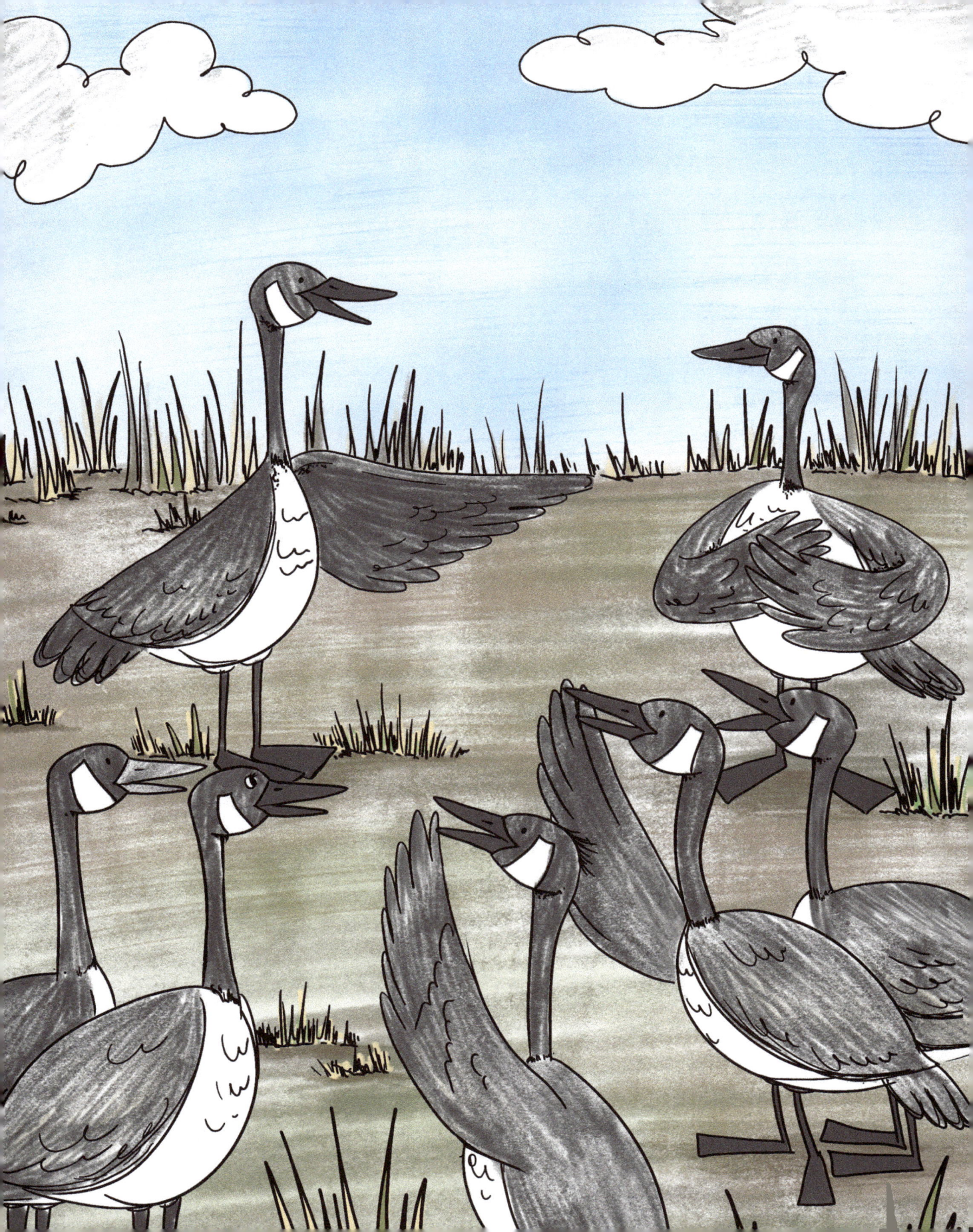

In the morning, the family flock flew high in the sky and into their *V* formation. Charley and Gus waved goodbye. It was a clear morning, and Charley and Gus stood side by side and watched until they could no longer see the family flock. It was nice to be together, and now, every day they would be together.

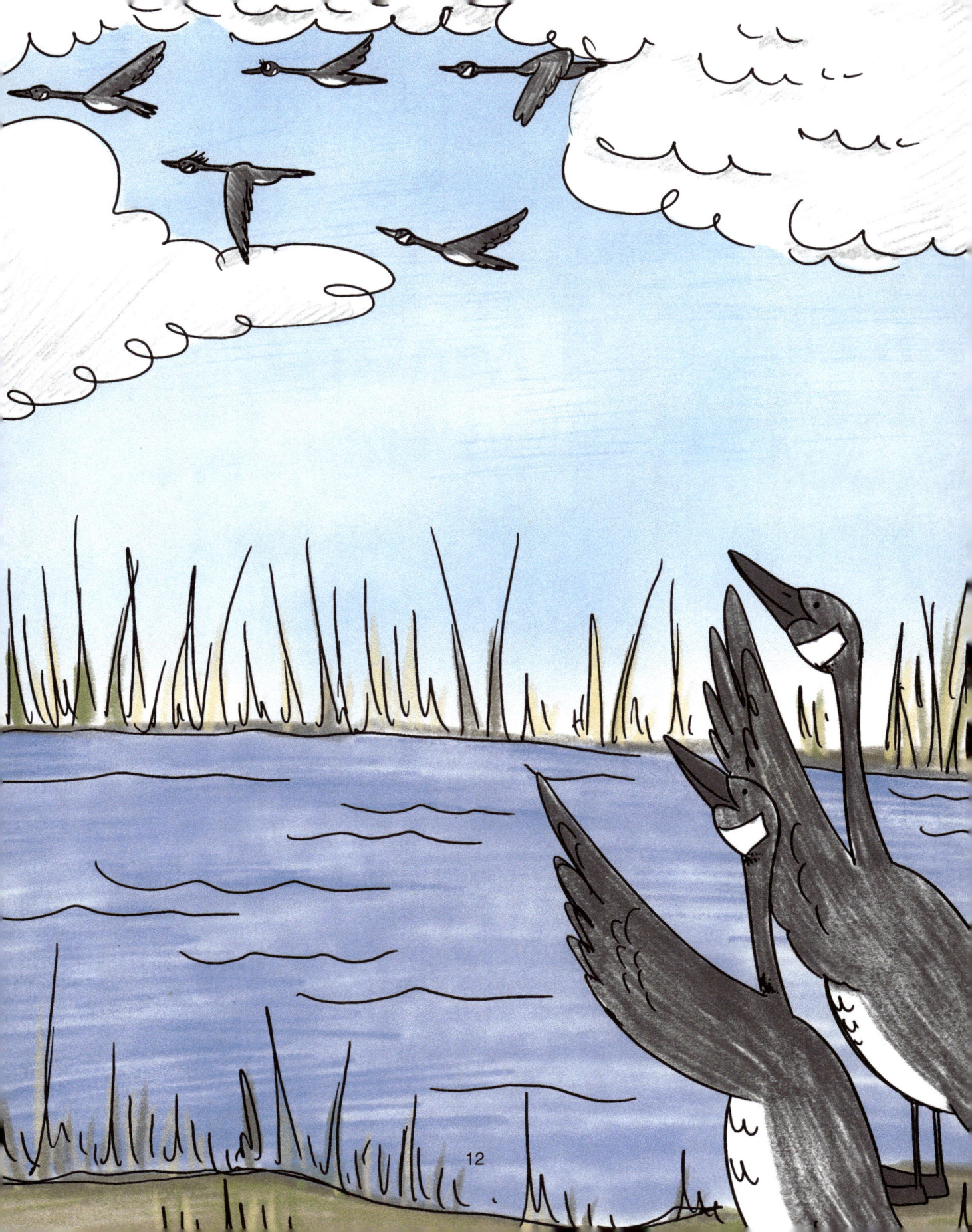

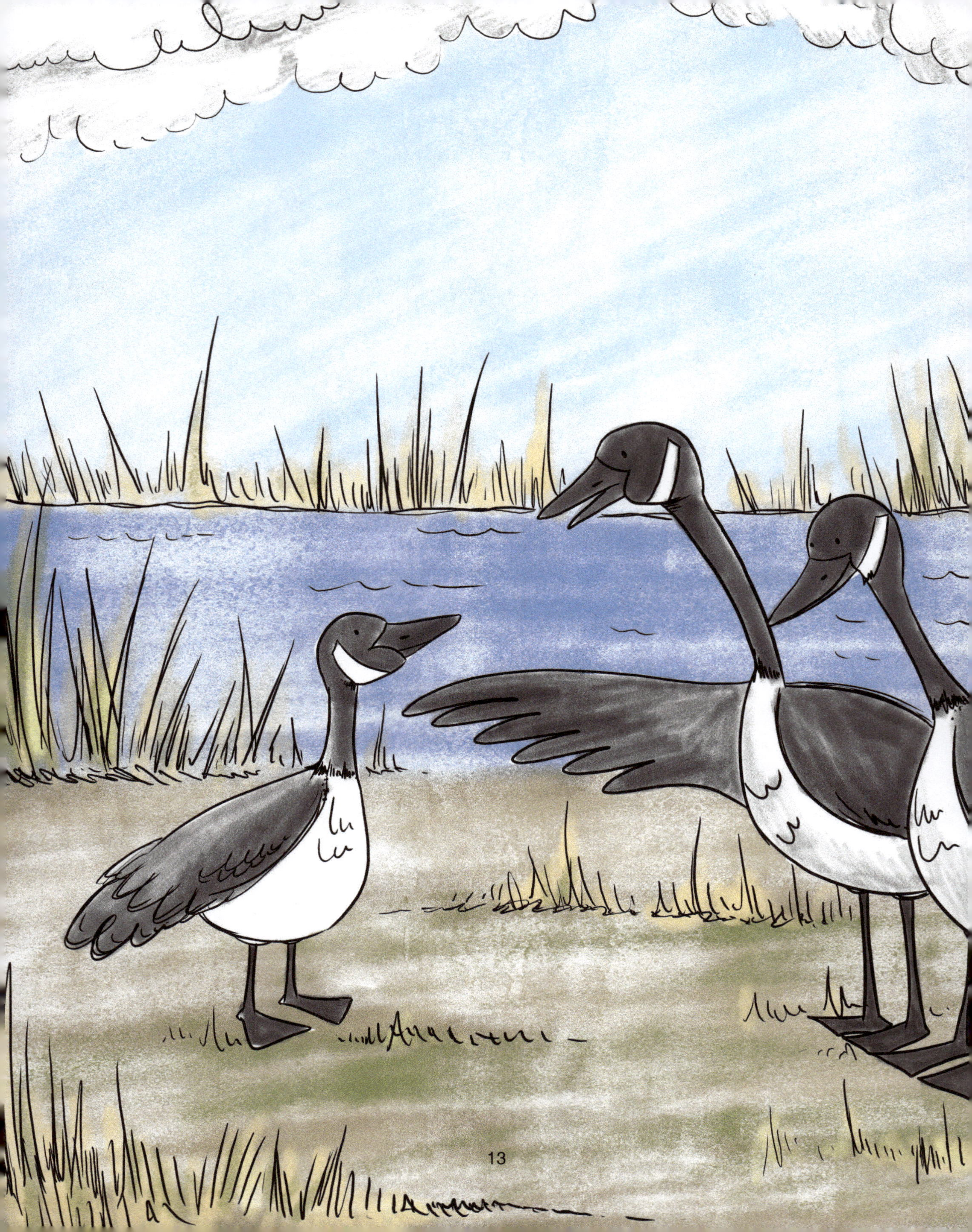

A few days later, Gus and Charley decided to take a walk. They walked all the way to the other side of the pond. Charley suddenly noticed something in the distance. "I think it is a Canada goose," said Charley. The little goose was different-looking with short wings and legs and a very short neck. Gus and Charley waddled over to the goose.

Gus said, "Hi, this is Charley, and I am Charley's big brother, Gus. We were taking a walk and saw you and wondered if anything was wrong or if you needed help."

The little goose told them her name was Charlotte and she was with her brother. "I was exhausted and dropped from my family's V formation." My brother left the V formation to check on me.

Geese are kindhearted, and if any goose withdraws from the V formation, another goose or several geese withdraw, too. They protect and care for the tired or injured goose.

Charlotte's brother saw Charley and Gus talking to his sister and quickly came over to make sure she was safe.

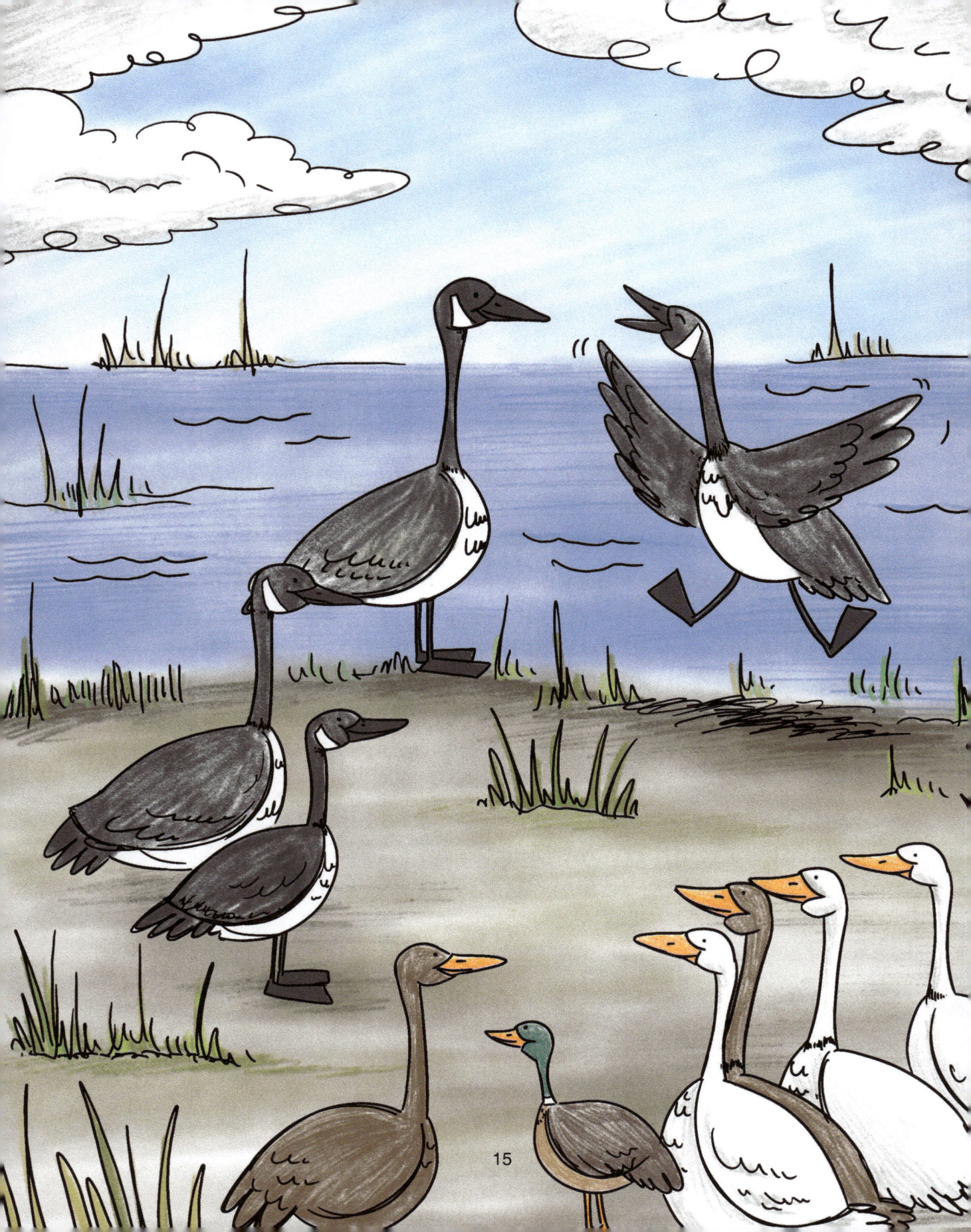

15

Gus and Charley told Charlotte's brother that they live here and invited the two geese to join them and their friends on the other side of the pond. The geese went with them tentatively.

The friends gathered around Charlotte and asked her why she was so little. Charlotte shrugged and said, "I was picked on a lot because I was a 'different-looking' goose, unlike all the other Canada geese. My wings and legs are short. It is hard for me to keep up with my family flock. I am not good at flying or swimming."

Her brother jumped into the conversation and said, "But she is the best at hide-and-seek. She also finds the best berries and grasses in the back of the bushes that no one else can find."

Charley confessed that he, too, was unlike his siblings and not good at flying or swimming either.

Gus said, "No worries. Look at us. Our friends are several domestic white geese, a few brown geese, and a mallard duck." Gus continued, "We are all different in size, color, shape, and personality. We do not care about differences. Differences are what make us special."

Charley started jumping up and down and said,

"Together, we can be different and still belong!
Together, we can be different and still belong!"

Charlotte and her brother decided to stay a few days to see if she would regain her strength. If she did, they would fly slowly and a few miles a day and return to their family flock. Unfortunately, Charlotte was not regaining her strength very fast. Gus, Charley, and their friends assured Charlotte's brother that he could rejoin his family flock and they would care for Charlotte through the winter. Charlotte agreed. The next day, Charlotte's brother said his goodbyes and wing-hugged Charlotte. Charlotte softly honked to her brother and said, "Tell the family I will be fine and we will see each other in the spring."

Gus and Charley and their friends liked Charlotte. She enjoyed the night sky talks by Charley. She liked that her new friends did not make fun of her and just liked her for whom she was. Charlotte really felt like she belonged. She especially loved being cared for by Gus. He was a kind, dependable, and compassionate good friend. Charlotte spent the winter with Gus, Charley, and their friends.

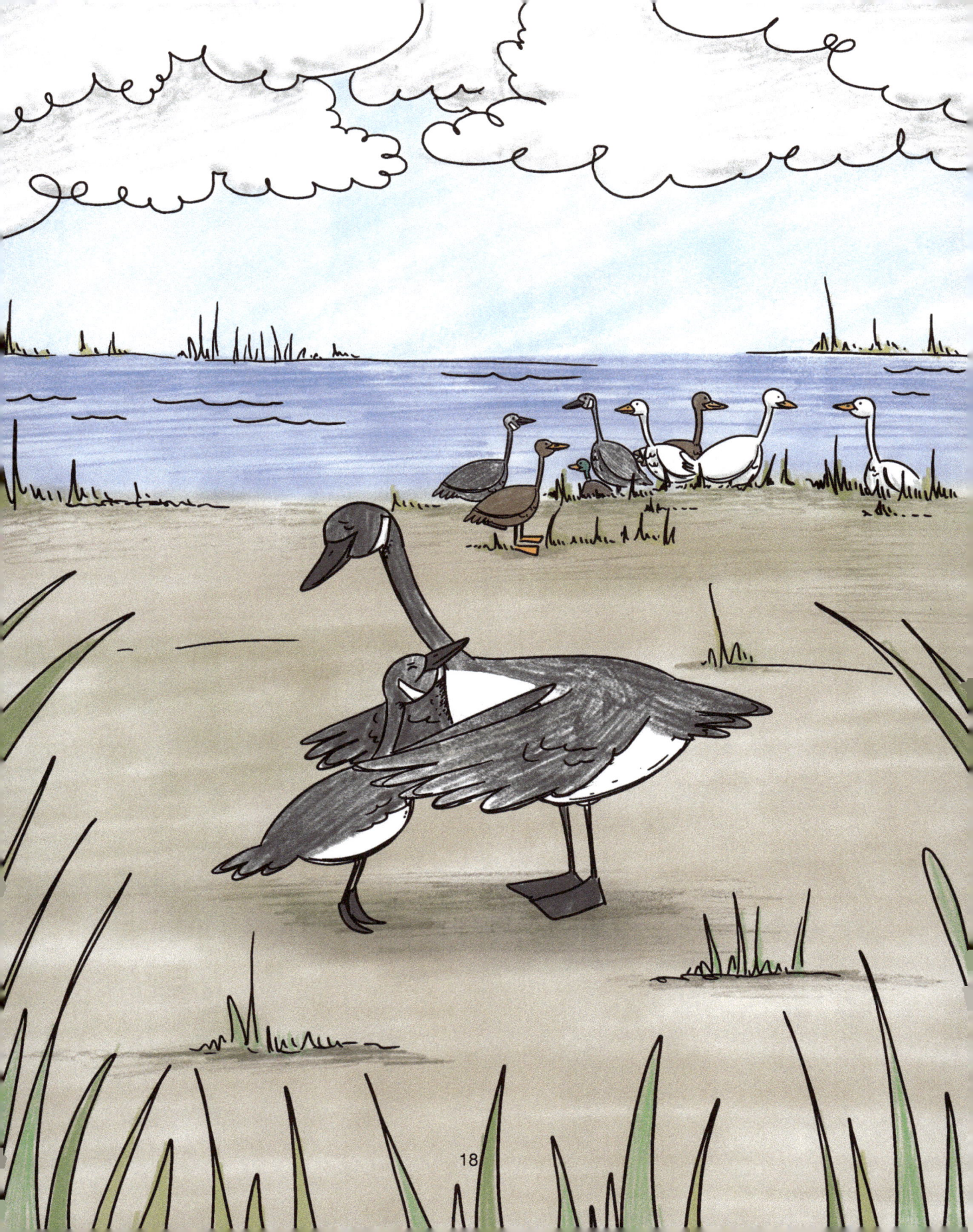

Mama Goose noticed that the days and nights were getting warmer. Winter was coming to an end. She gathered the flock together and said, "In the morning we are flying back to our nesting site. Of course, we will be stopping to visit Charley and Gus." Everyone was happy except Sammy.

Sammy, with his neck hung low, looked up and asked, "May I bring my new friend along?"

Josie said, "What friend?"

"Well," said Sammy, "one afternoon while I was flying around, I met a mourning dove that could fly almost as fast as I can. Sometimes, we raced each other, and other times we enjoyed playing tag. Her name is Betty. She is so much fun, and we have become the best of friends."

The mourning dove is considered *one* of the fastest backyard birds. They can fly about forty miles per hour and have reached speeds of fifty-five miles per hour.

Sammy asked again, "May I bring her along?"

Father Goose looked at Mama Goose, and she gave a favorable nod. Father Goose smiled and said, "Yes, Sammy, you can invite Betty to join us. Betty can have a special place and fly right behind me in the center of the *V* formation."

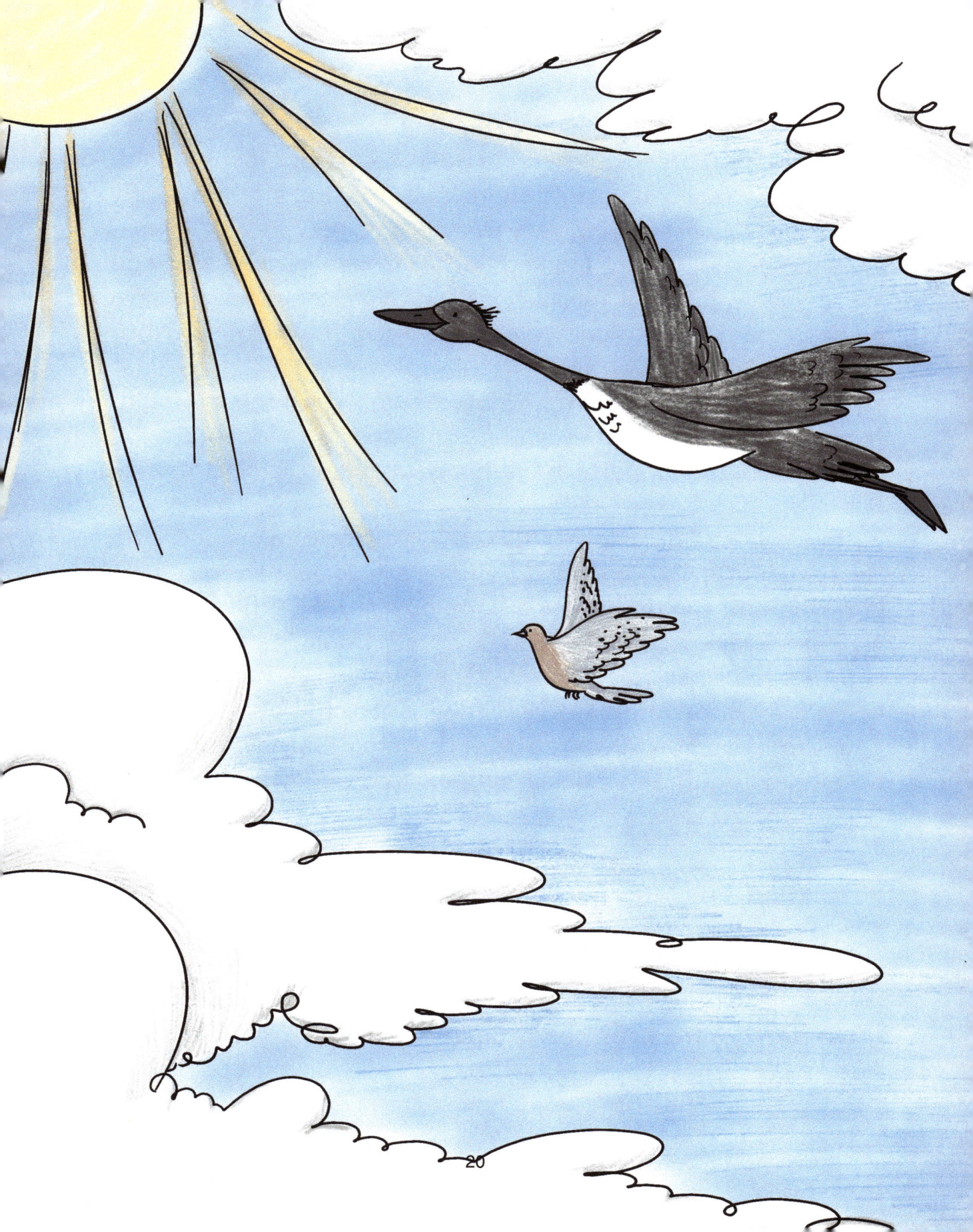

Sammy flew off to quickly find Betty to ask her if she would like to join their family flock and fly to their nesting site. Betty, flying nearby, saw Sammy flying very fast toward her.

Sammy said, "Betty, I asked Father Goose, and he said I could invite you to join our family flock, and you could have a special place in our *V* formation. We are leaving in the morning. What do you think, Betty?"

Betty, thinking for a few minutes, said, "Yes, I think I would like to go with you. I have always wanted to see new places."

Sammy was happy to have his best friend joining the family flock.

Sammy and Betty flew to tell the family flock. Sammy introduced Betty to his family. He said, "Over there is Josie with the beautiful big eyes and Gertie with the light-colored bill. I have two more siblings, Charley and Gus, and they live in Charley's place. Charley is unlike his siblings; he has autism. Gus enjoys helping him and being his big brother. We visit them every fall and spring for a couple of days. You will get to meet them too." Sammy smiled. "When we all get together, Charley gets excited and starts jumping up and down and says,

'Together, we can be different and still belong!
Together, we can be different and still belong!'"

Morning came quickly. The family flock and their new family member, Betty, formed the *V* formation and left their wintering grounds. They were excited to leave and eager to see Charley and Gus.

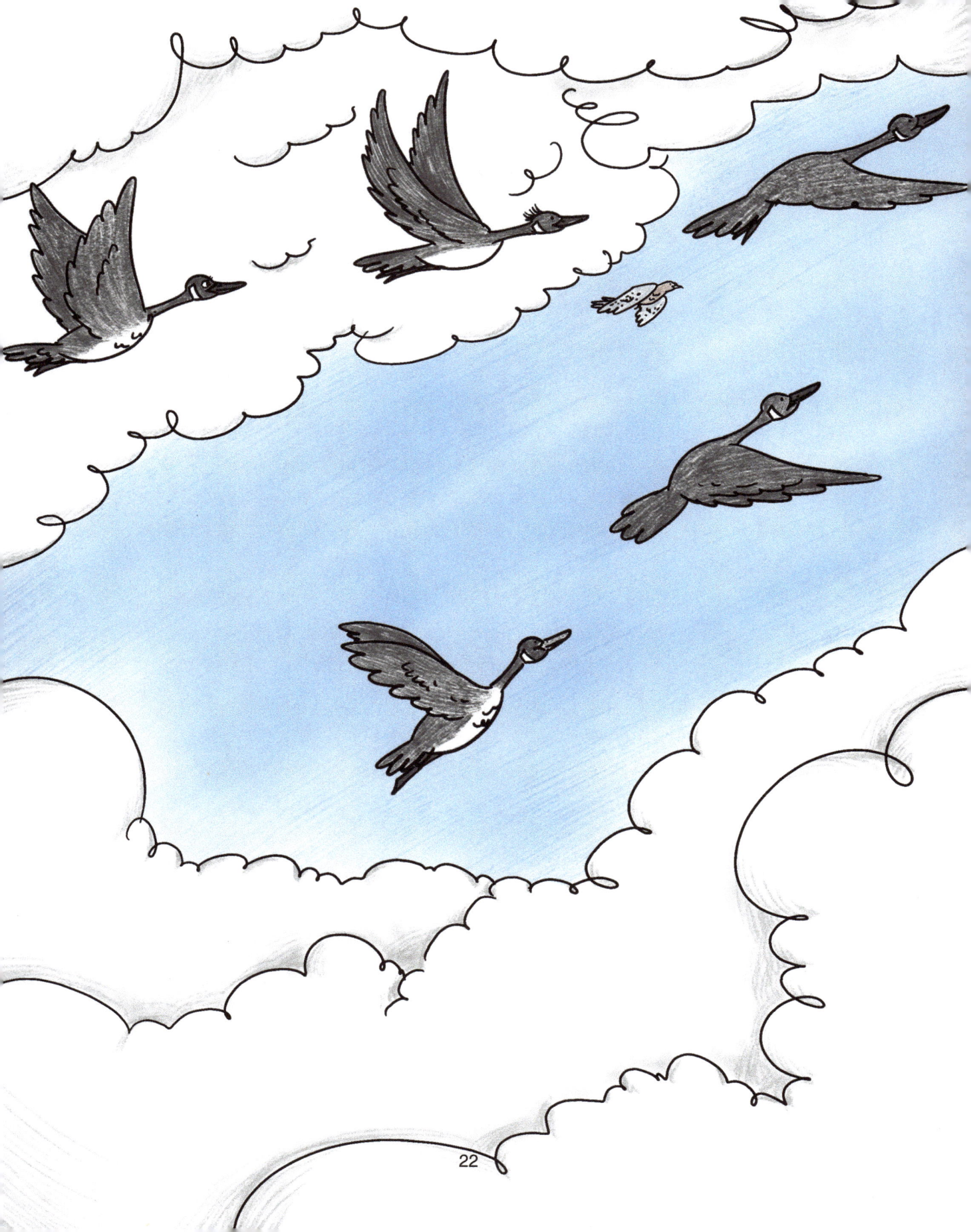

With spring coming to Charley's place, Charlotte told Gus she felt the desire to migrate to her nesting site and find her family flock. "I like it here, and you have all been so nice to me," she said, "but I feel like I should rejoin my family." Gus was sad because he liked her a lot.

Later that day, Gus and Charlotte talked and talked about her returning to her family and how much they would miss each other. He pleaded with her to not leave until his family flock came. Gus wanted her to meet Mama Goose and Father Goose, Josie, Gertie, and Sammy. "You may want to join their *V* formation until you find your family." Charlotte agreed to wait and decide about leaving until after she met Gus and Charley's family flock.

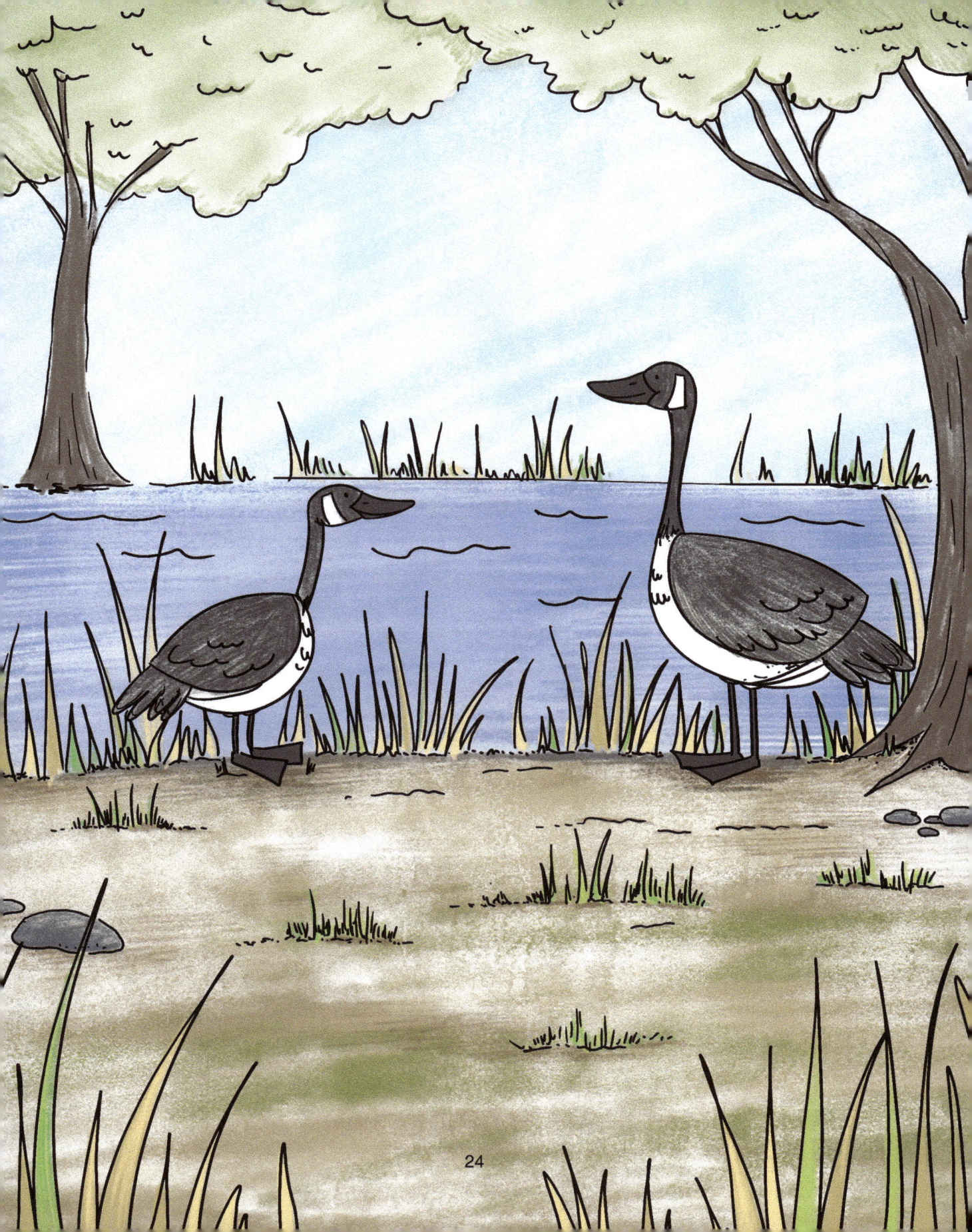

Charley, looking up into the sky while covering his ears, saw that it was filled with many noisy *V* formations of Canada geese traveling north. He shouted, "Hey, everyone, come here!" Charley saw a *V* formation coming closer and closer and lower and lower toward them. "It is our family flock and, I think, a mourning dove." Charley was good at noticing details, and he knew he would spot them first!

Family wing tip hugs were shared. Sammy told everyone that Betty was his best friend. Charley got excited and started jumping up and down and said,

"Together, we can be different and still belong!
Together, we can be different and still belong!"

Gus smiled and said, "I have a new friend too. Her name is Charlotte."

Charley quickly started to chant over and over, "Gus likes Charlotte! Gus likes Charlotte!"

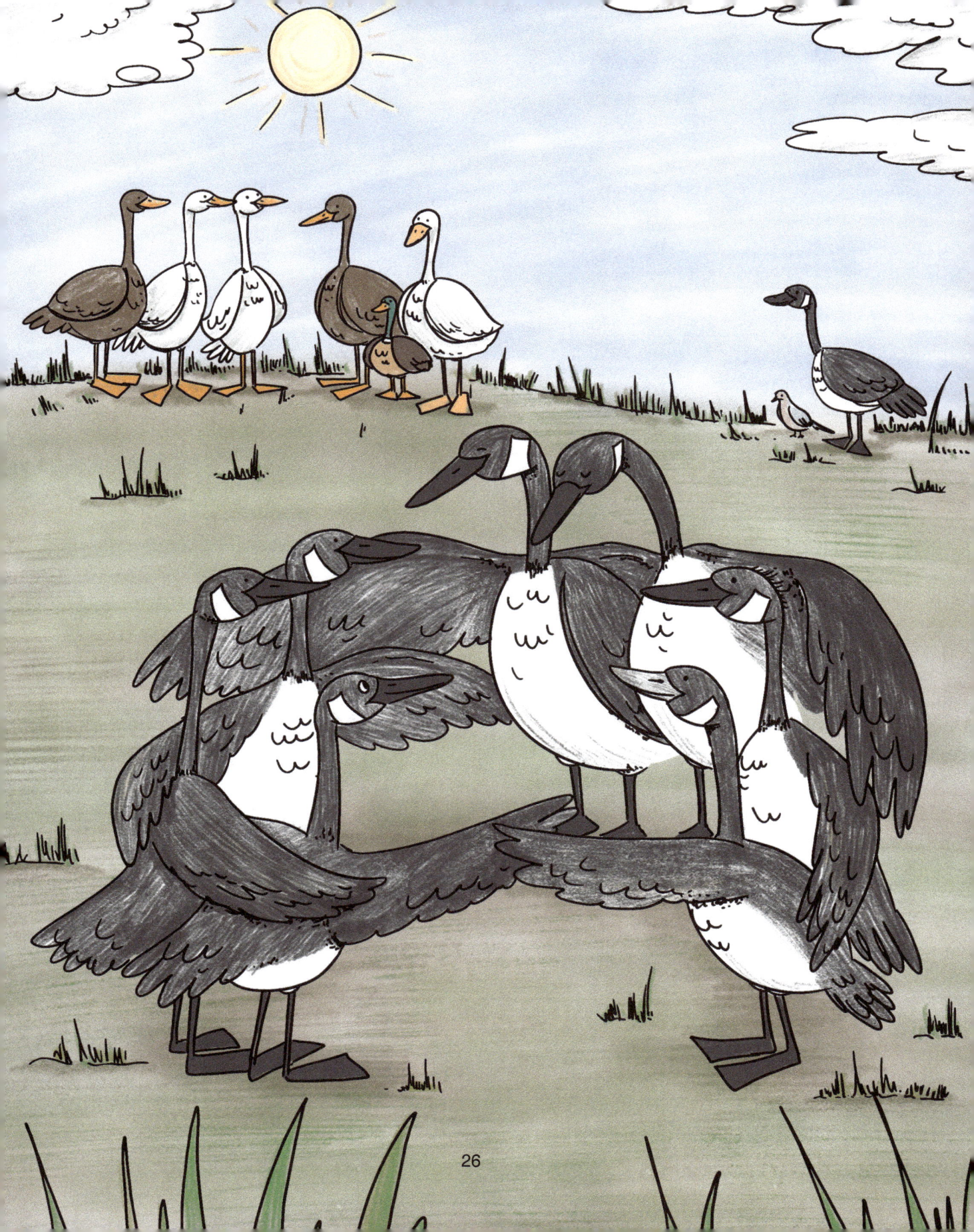

Gus told the family flock that they met Charlotte on the other side of the pond. "She had dropped from her family's *V* formation. As time passed, Charlotte was not recovering very quickly and needed more time. Charlotte stayed with us through the winter. She is ready now to return to her family flock and may want to join your *V* formation until she locates her family." Gus, looking over at Charlotte, smiled and said, "Or maybe she will stay here with Charley and me!" He was hopeful as he had grown very fond of Charlotte.

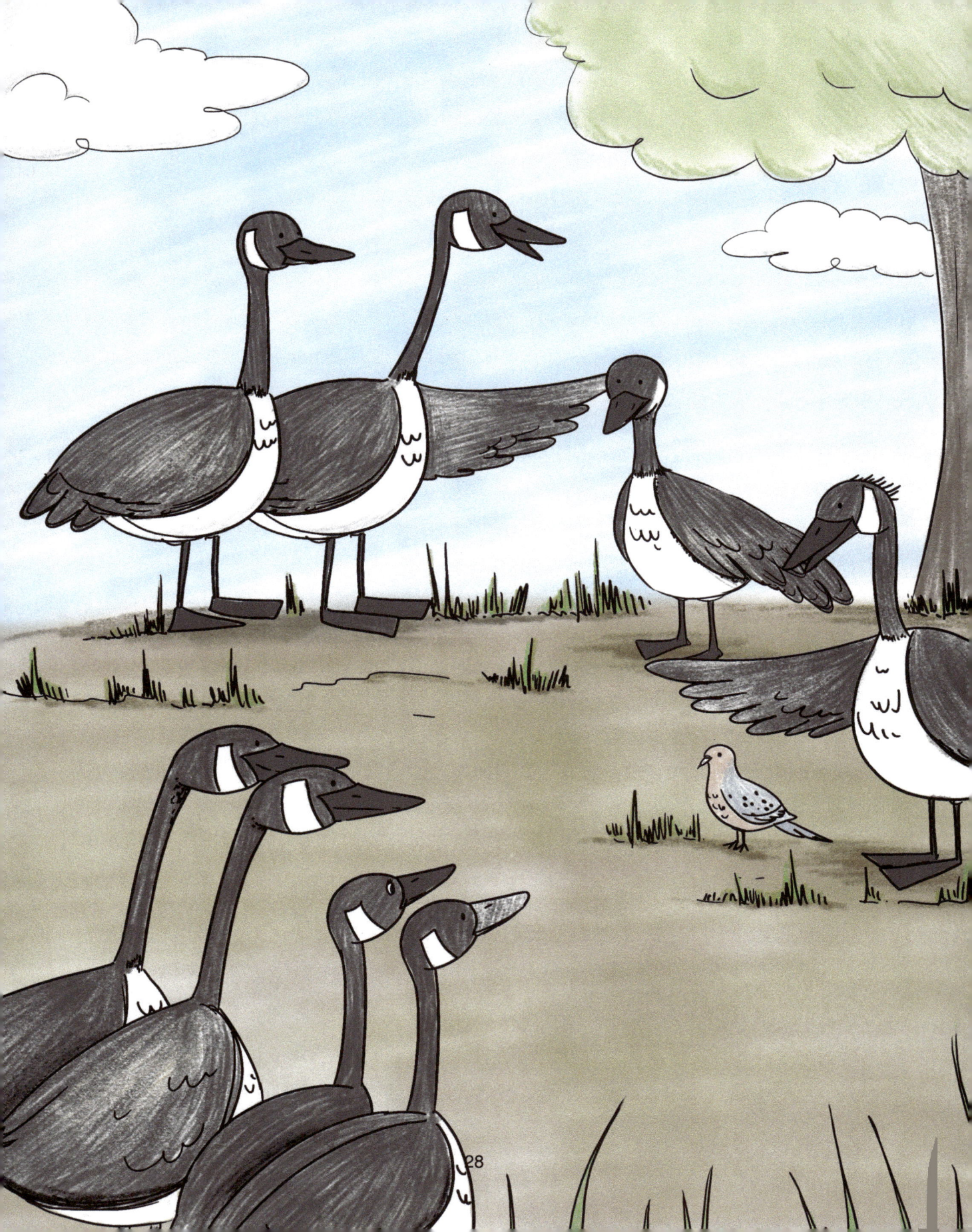

28

After spending a few days together, Mama Goose said, "It is time to go. We will leave in the morning. Charlotte, you are welcome to join us."

Charlotte thanked her and said, "I'll think about it."

Mama Goose instructed everyone to get a good night's sleep because tomorrow was the day to start the journey north back to their nesting site.

Charlotte really liked Gus and felt accepted by Charley and their friends. It was the best winter she had ever had. It was the first time she felt she was able to be herself and was loved even though she was different. Charlotte waddled over to Gus and covered his eyes with her wings and said, "Guess what?" She whispered in his ear, "I'm going to stay with you." Gus was so excited. He honked and honked as loud as he could. Everyone knew this meant that Charlotte had decided to stay with Gus and Charley.

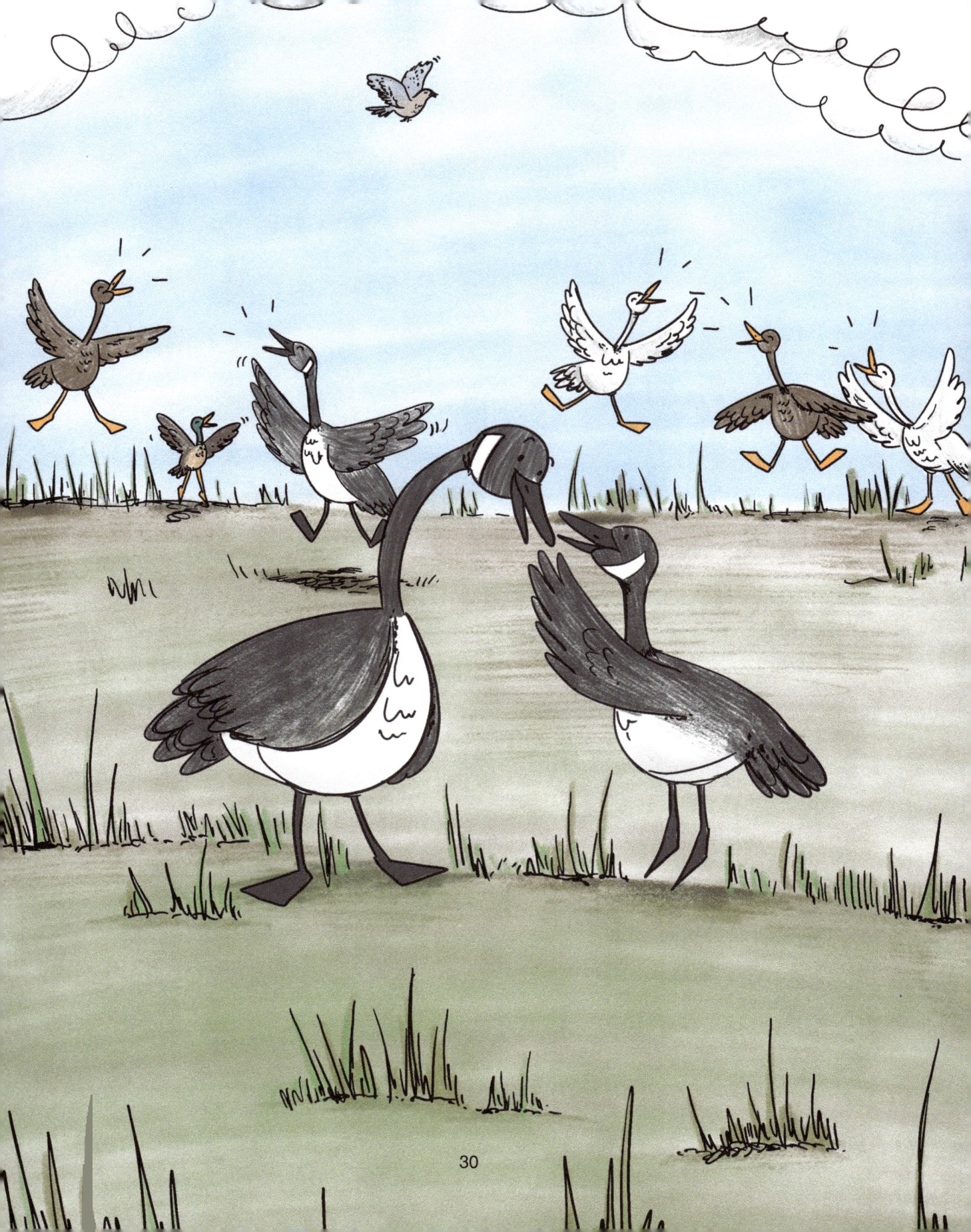

Gus and Charlotte spent a lot of time together. Charley was always tagging along. One warm spring morning on the edge of the pond, Gus and Charlotte started to build a nest in the rushes. Charley helped build the nest by collecting grasses. Soon three eggs were laid. Charlotte incubated the eggs in her nest for about thirty days. Gus and Charley and their friends watched over Charlotte and the three eggs. When the goslings started to hatch, Gus honked loudly for all to come. He was proud of becoming a father just like Father Goose.

They all listened to the cracking noise, and soon, out from the eggs popped three little heads. The goslings climbed out of the shells. They looked like puffballs.

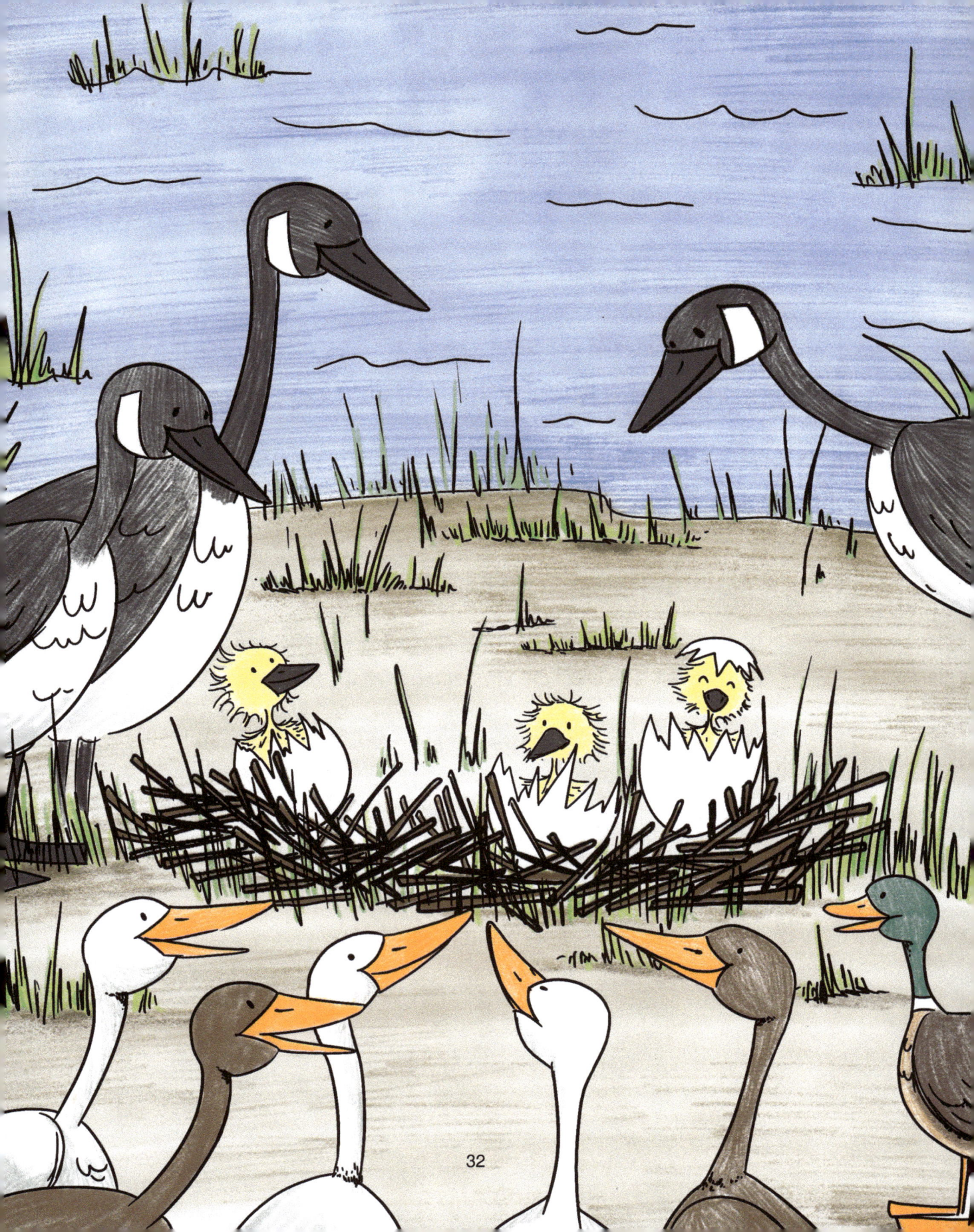

Gus said, "Wait until Mama Goose and Father Goose, Josie, Gertie, Sammy, and Betty come in the fall. They will see our three new family members. They will be so surprised!"

Charley started jumping up and down and said,

"Together, we can be different and still belong!
Together, we can be different and still belong!"

Gus, spreading out his wings, said, "Come here, everyone, for a big family hug!"

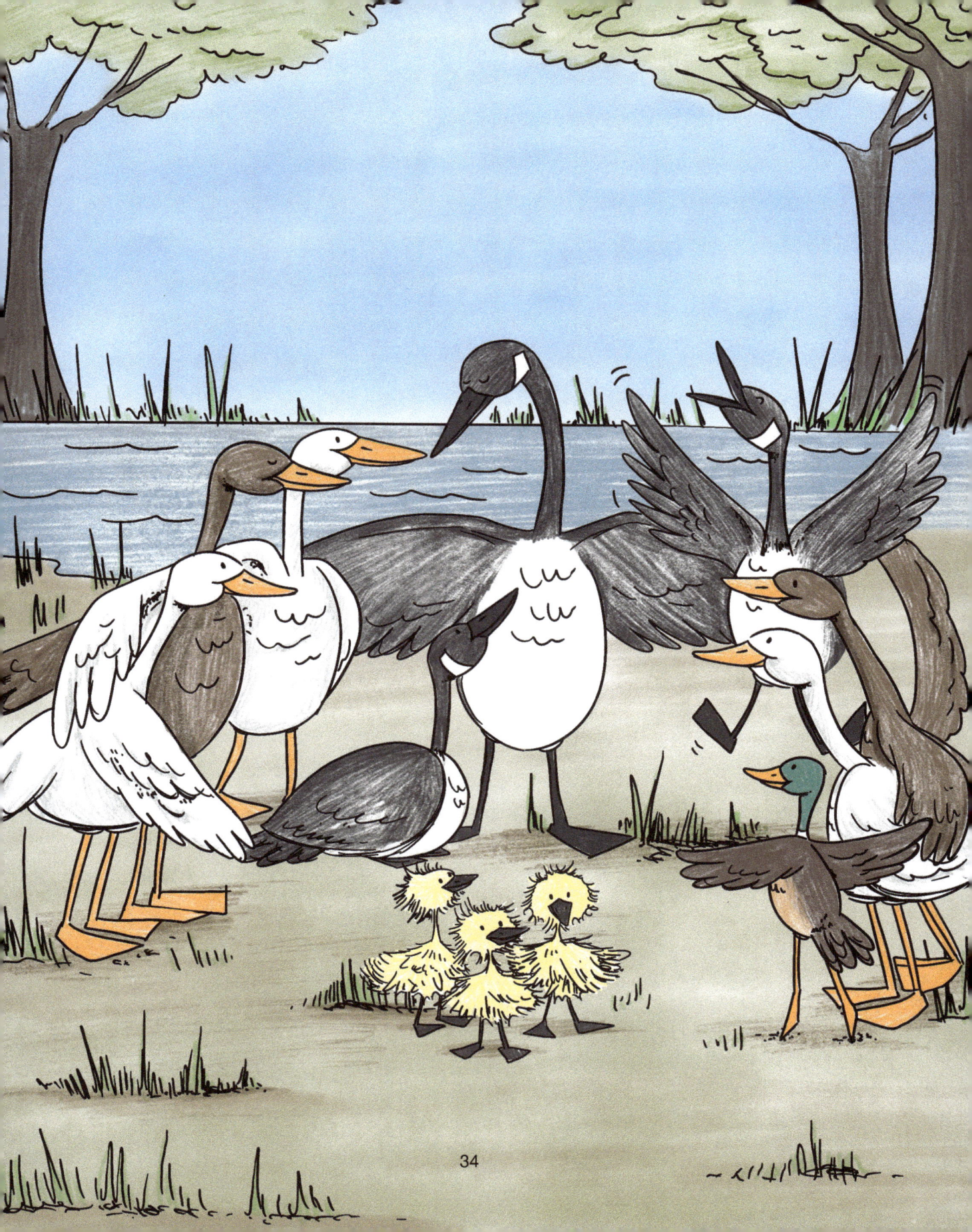

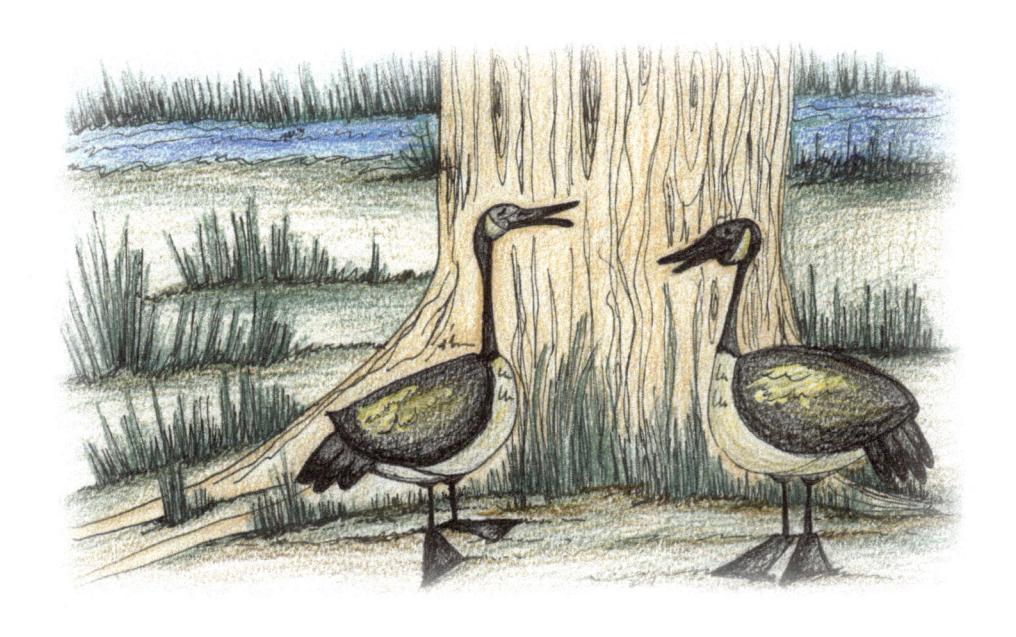

For Our Readers
Discussion Questions

1. How are you like Gus?

2. Do you have a sibling or a friend like Gus?

3. What is your favorite part of the story?

4. Have you ever had a secret?

5. What do the words "Together, we can be different and still belong" mean to you?

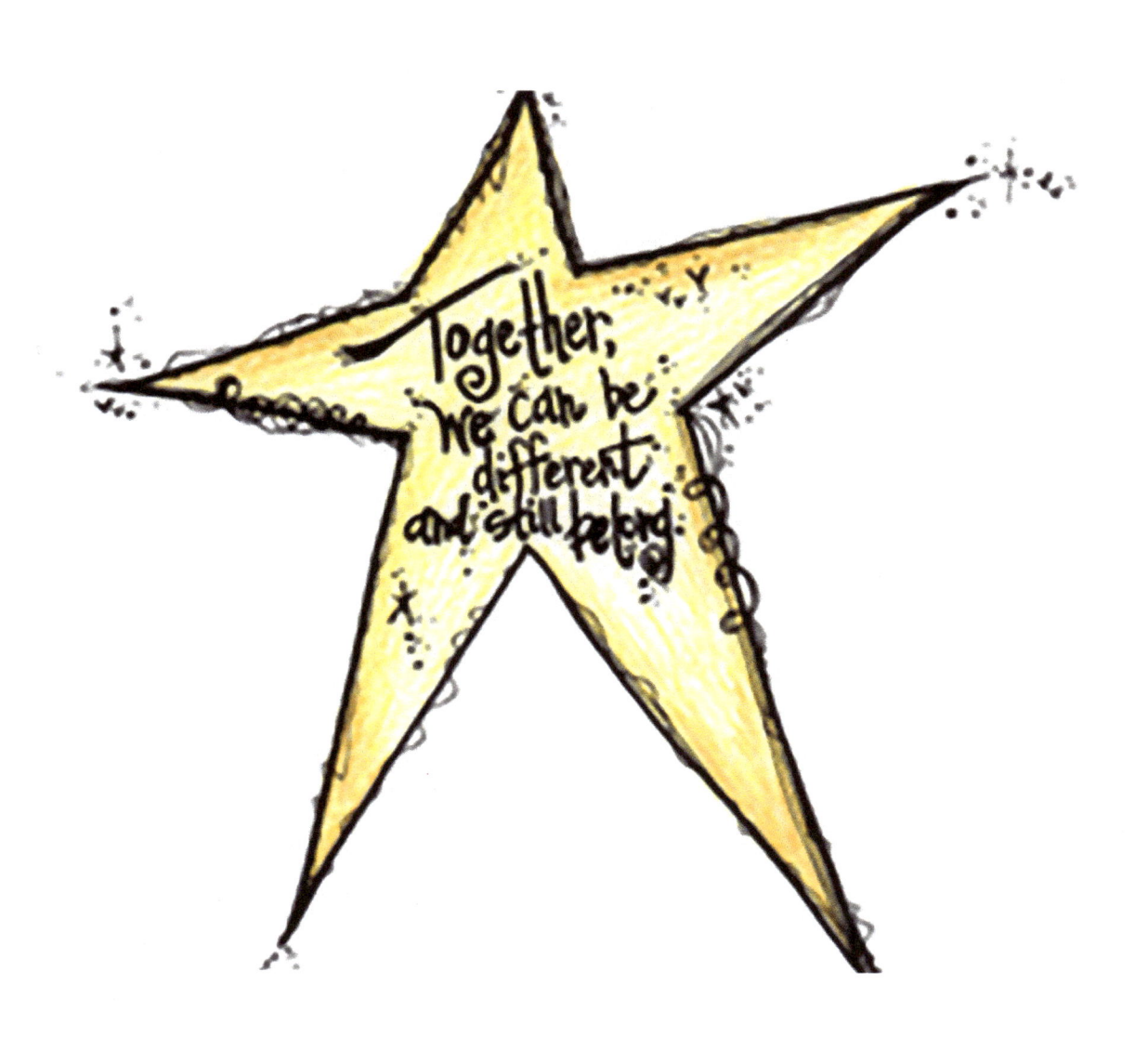

About the Author

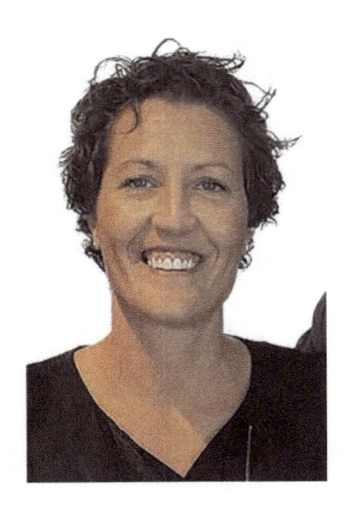

Morghan E. Bosch, EdD, is an associate professor of special education at Barton College, North Carolina. She teaches courses in autism, exceptionalities, and assists students in research endeavors. Dr. Bosch has written several books and articles on special education topics. She has presented at many national conferences on exceptionalities with the message "Together, we can be different and still belong." The series *Embracing Differences* is a thought-provoking opportunity to promote awareness, understanding, and acceptance of individual differences.

CPSIA information can be obtained
at www.ICGtesting.com
Printed in the USA
LVHW010720140523
746939LV00007B/107